Medical Emergencies

A Guide for Navigating the Healthcare System

Peggy Calestro

Copyright © 2020 Peggy Calestro
All rights reserved
First Edition

PAGE PUBLISHING, INC.
Conneaut Lake, PA

First originally published by Page Publishing 2020

ISBN 978-1-6624-0795-6 (pbk)
ISBN 978-1-6624-0796-3 (digital)

Printed in the United States of America

Contents

PREFACE 1

HOSPITALS 5

    Introduction 6

    What You Need to Know 7

    Hospitalists 8

    Treatment Plan 10

    Hospital Jargon 10

    Medication Drift 13

    Take Care of Yourself 14

    Leaving the Hospital: Going Home 15

  Leaving the Hospital: Going to an Aftercare Facility 16

SURGERY 17

  Advice for the Waiting Room 20

  After Surgery 20

AFTERCARE 23

  Home Care 24

  Home-Based Nursing or Therapeutic Services 26

    Frequency of Home Visits by the Healthcare Professional 26

  Nonmedical Home-Based Care 27

  Rehabilitation Facilities 31

  Assisted Living 34

    Cost of Care 36

    Neglect and Abuse 40

FAMILY MEMBERS, FRIENDS, AND NEIGHBORS 42

  Beyond the Casserole 45

  Helping with Medications 46

    Mail, Pets, and Housekeeping 46

    Give Caregivers a Break 47

LEGAL AND FINANCIAL CONCERNS 48

    Medical Power of Attorney (Also Called
    Power of Attorney for Healthcare or Durable
    Power of Attorney for Healthcare) 50

    Living Will (Also Known as Advanced
    Healthcare Directive) 50

    Financial Power of Attorney 51

    Guardianship 51

    Will 52

    Medical Bills 53

SUMMARY 55

PREFACE

My experience with hospital bureaucracies began more than twenty years ago.

I was sitting in the crowded lobby of a regional cancer center near the registration desk. Two elderly women who could have been sisters were answering questions posed by the clerk. Her final question was, "Next of kin?" I watched as the two sisters visibly recoiled, grabbed each other's hands, and considered the ramifications of that question.

After they were seated, I approached the desk and quietly asked the clerk if there might be another way to phrase the last question—something like "Is there someone we can call in case of an emergency?" or "Whom shall we contact if we have questions?"

The clerk smiled apologetically and said she was required to ask the questions exactly as they appeared on the form. I asked how we could change the form. She didn't know but gave me a customer–comment card to complete.

That would be the first of dozens of suggestions and complaints I wrote on the customer–comment form over my yearlong course of treatment. I put most in the drop box, even hand-delivered a few to the hospital administrator's office, but I never received a response. Years later, I discovered this is not unique to American hospitals.*

---

* A 2017 study of United Kingdom hospitals found that "making changes based on patient feedback is a complex, multi-tiered process and not something that ward staff can simply 'do'… Despite the wealth of feedback now available to

As far as I know, none of my suggestions was implemented. The flavored-coffee kiosk, spewing its overwhelming hazelnut odor down the hallway corridor, remained adjacent to the chemotherapy wing. The people buying coffee there were all hospital staff, but there are thousands of ex-patients who will forever associate the smell of hazelnut coffee with the nausea of chemotherapy.

This guidebook, however, deals not with my cancer treatment but with my family's and friends' decades of experience in the healthcare system: surgeries; multiple hospitalizations; inpatient and outpatient physical, speech and occupational therapy; home healthcare providers; rehabilitation and assisted-care facilities; and the numerous physicians, nurses, techs and support staff delivering this care in a variety of settings.

My purpose in writing this book is to help families and friends of people who have suffered an unexpected catastrophic medical event—an event that changes the lives not only of the patients themselves but of those around them.

My hope is that our individual and collective experiences will be useful to others who find it necessary to navigate a complex healthcare system during extremely stressful times.

---

heathcare services, there is little evidence that this feedback has led to improvement in the quality of healthcare." (Soc Sci Med. 2017 Apr; 178: 19–27)

HOSPITALS

Introduction

HOSPITALS ARE INVALUABLE in helping patients survive medical crises. They employ a variety of healthcare workers who have entered the profession because they are committed to helping others and are well trained, licensed, and certified to work in medical settings. Hospitals have numerous specialists and departments available to diagnose and treat a variety of illnesses and complications.

That said, hospitals are not good places to relax and heal.

They're noisy, germy, and uncomfortable. Machines beep and hum, wires are everywhere, room temperatures may be too cold or too hot. Although there have been advances in reducing infections, even the best of hospitals have outbreaks of MRSA, staph, strep, norovirus, and flu. Staff are often overworked and underpaid.

The politics and management charts of hospital staff make it difficult to communicate with the people who are actually making decisions on your patient's care: physicians and nonclinical administrators. The professionals who provide direct care to patients (nurses, techs, social workers, physical therapists) often are not authorized to determine what tests or medications are needed, how to interpret test results, or when a patient can go home.

Instead, those decisions are made by physicians, whose actual time with the patient may be very limited. Physicians often visit patients during the early morning hours, long before family members arrive, or when the patient may be too groggy to understand or to relay what was said. The result is that someone other than the physician (a nurse, social worker, or hospitalist) has to explain the course of care to the family and patient. This secondhand communication system does not allow the family to ask questions or to explore other options with the physician.

The situation gets even more complicated when the patient is under the care of multiple departments, such as cardiology, neurology, and urology. It's no secret there is a pecking order to these specialties and that doctors do not necessarily coordinate care across departments.

As a result, family and friends must become informed and vocal advocates for the patient.

What You Need to Know

The following questions will help the family obtain information and gain some control over the patient's care.

Which physician is primarily responsible for the patient's care? The answer to this question may change over the course of a patient's stay in the hospital. For instance, a patient who is admitted for cardiac surgery (cardiology) but suffers a stroke and kidney complications as a result of the surgery (neurology, urology), may be under the care of specialists from three departments. Each of these specialists may recommend different tests, medications, therapy, and length of hospital stay.

Families must continue to ask, "Who has the ultimate authority over our patient's care?" Without a specific answer to this question, patients can languish in the hospital for many more days than necessary before being allowed to leave.

Keep a notebook of medical contacts. Record the name, phone number (office and pager) of the primary decision-making physician, as well as any colleagues who are covering patient care during weekend or vacation absences. Keep all this information in one place, like a notebook or folder.

Hospitalists

The Joint Commission on Accreditation of Hospitals requires that a patient advocate be available at all times in a hospital. The position of hospitalist fills that requirement.

This relatively new medical specialty was added to the healthcare team to serve as liaisons between medical staff and families, helping to interpret test results and answer questions. Hospitalists are medical doctors, usually general internists, whose specialty is caring for patients in hospitals.

Hospitalists often fill the role of the patient's primary physician, whose schedule does not allow daily visits to see hospitalized patients or to meet with their families. In many inpatient healthcare facilities, hospitalists play an important role in determining when your patient can be released.

Hospitalists function as information technology specialists whose job is to assemble large amounts of objective data (results of lab tests, patient's vital signs, clinical notes), synthesize these data, and communicate the conclusions. It's your office's "IT guy" in a healthcare setting.

Hospitalists arrive at the scene with some disadvantages. Patients and families haven't chosen them; they are assigned. As such, they have no personal knowledge of the patient or family other than what's contained on multiple screens of the patient's computer file.

Because it's a new specialty, and many hospitalists are newly graduated doctors, they may rank low on the hierarchy of physicians. This can create a perfect storm for patients and their families. As relatively new team members, hospitalists often must defer to the opinions of attending physicians from different specialties who outrank them in experience and tenure and may have opposing recommendations on a patient's release date or follow-up care. This can create delays and confusion.

If your family is unhappy with the hospitalist assigned to your patient, you should ask for another. Alternately, you can hire your own independent patient advocate through an outside organization such as the AdvoConnection.

Treatment Plan

Families should ask for a copy of the treatment plan twenty-four hours after the patient is admitted. This plan describes what the healthcare team is doing for symptom X, for symptom Y, and so on, as well as the expected outcomes.

Ask healthcare staff to explain anything you don't understand. Remember: It's your right to have this information and to understand it.

Ask if any parts of the treatment plan could be done on an outpatient basis. This information will give you a better understanding of the healthcare team's focus and how the patient's progress toward those goals will be measured.

Hospital Jargon[*]

Remember that families have a right to honest and easy-to-understand medical and treatment information about the patient. Most healthcare professionals avoid using complicated medical terms when talking with patients and families. It's always a good idea to have someone in the

---

[*] A recent study published in the <u>British Dental Journal</u> found that more than 30 percent of English-speaking patients were unable to define simple medical terms such as lesion and benign. Thirty percent of English-speaking survey participants thought a biopsy was a confirmation of cancer (Ayers Career College).

family taking notes when it comes to test results and the expected course of treatment.

Our family was fortunate to have my daughter, a social worker who has worked in hospitals for more than a decade, and a family friend who is a physician to ask more technical questions. Both understand medical terminology and the process by which hospitals make decisions on a patient's care.

One important phrase hospitals use is <u>differential diagnosis</u>. *Wikipedia* defines this as the process of differentiating between two or more conditions which share similar symptoms: identifying a specific disease and eliminating others. The example used is, "Acute bronchitis could be a differential diagnosis in evaluating a cough, even if the final diagnosis is a common cold."

During a hospitalization for my husband, I was amazed at how much more information we received when my daughter requested his differential diagnosis. By asking this question, families will get a lot more detailed answers on what symptoms the team is looking at and the diagnosis toward which they're leaning. The differential diagnosis creates a much better understanding of the need for all the tests, monitoring devices, procedures, and multiple healthcare staff.

After hospital admission, patients and families should ask, "How soon can we leave?" This answer will be based on objective (measurable) medical criteria, such as a certain blood pressure number, a certain kidney creatine level, ability to stand and walk after surgery, etc. This information will help patients and families keep track of patient progress toward getting released.

Insurance coverage also may dictate the patient's length of stay, or at least what expenses will be covered by the policy. Hospitals employ liaisons to work with insurance companies to determine if the patient is making sufficient progress to warrant a continued (policy-paid) hospital stay. Insurance companies also must approve medical procedures and medications.

Most hospitals are not interested in keeping patients beyond what is medically necessary, but families should be clear about how doctors will decide whether it's time to be discharged.

If the patient is under the care of physicians from different departments, this decision can be delayed for longer than necessary. There may be medical disagreements among doctors, but more likely, it will be departmental politics or bureaucratic pecking order that dictates when a decision can be made.

We once waited eight days on an inpatient unit until consensus could be reached on follow-up care. In our case, my husband's physical and mental well-bring deteriorated considerably during this wait. Because of indecision and interdepartmental politics, he was caught in a kind of bureaucratic limbo and ultimately left the hospital much sicker than when he arrived. One person I know became so angry with the lack of a specific date for his mother's release that hospital security threatened to have him arrested.

Medication Drift

Chances are the list of medications for your patient will grow with every hospital or rehabilitation facility stay. My term for this is "medication drift." Here's an example:

Let's say the patient is admitted to the hospital with high blood pressure, which physicians get under control immediately. But the patient develops a sore shoulder from lying in a hospital bed, so Dr. X prescribes a mild muscle relaxer; in a day or so, this medication creates a stomach ache, so Dr. Y prescribes antacid/anti-nausea medicine. But no one takes him off the original muscle relaxer or antacid when the patient goes home. When he was discharged from one hospital stay, my husband had accumulated a list of twenty-two current medications. After our questioning, his physician and pharmacist later reduced the list to only five that he needed.

In addition to your family physician, your best guide to avoid unnecessary medications is your family's pharmacist. The hospital or rehab center will give you a list of medications when the patient is discharged. Ask your local pharmacist to review that list for possible drug interactions, side effects, best times of day to administer (with or without food), any food or supplement interactions, etc.

See the FAMILY MEMBERS, FRIENDS, AND NEIGHBORS section for more advice on medications.

Take Care of Yourself

Families often forget to take care of themselves when a loved one is in the hospital. We have a tendency to gather in a group and sit and wait during the patient's surgery, or to gather in a group and sit and wait for updates from medical staff during the patient's hospital stay. But all this sitting and waiting can take its toll, both physically and emotionally.

My advice is to take time off from these vigils. Find opportunities to go home, to rest if possible, and to recharge. If the surgery will take several hours, or if the patient is stable in a hospital room, use this time to get some relief from the sitting and waiting. You'll need all of your strength and clear thinking in the coming days when your patient comes home or goes to another facility. Don't feel guilty when you leave the hospital. Qualified medical staff are there to monitor your patient's care while you're taking care of yourself, and they have your phone number if they need to contact you.

If the hospital is not in your hometown, ask the social worker assigned to your patient if there are nearby or partner hotels with discounts or other comfort items that cater to hospital families.

Leaving the Hospital: Going Home

Before bringing the patient home from the hospital, you might find it helpful to read the section on "Home Care." It offers some tips on how to determine if home is the best alternative for the patient.

Patients will receive a detailed list of prescriptions and follow-up instructions when they are discharged from the hospital. In addition to this information, families should always ask:

Is there anything we should look for that would require a trip to the emergency room? Answers to this question might include a high fever, elevated blood pressure, inability to urinate, or other signs of an infection.

Note: The length of hospital stay and the procedures and medications can cause patients to be weak, groggy, and nauseated. Keep plastic bags, paper towels, and wet wipes in your car so you'll be prepared for the trip home.

Leaving the Hospital: Going to an Aftercare Facility

If the patient requires some kind of medically supervised care after being hospitalized, see the next sections covering AFTERCARE.

If the patient must return to the hospital at a later date for surgery, go to the SURGERY section.

SURGERY

It's ALMOST IMPOSSIBLE for a family to prepare for unexpected surgery when a patient is admitted through the hospital's emergency room.

But if your family has advance notice of the upcoming surgery, here are some things to consider:

Determine if there is an alternative to surgery. Any surgical procedure—even a simple tooth extraction—is an invasive trauma to the body. Depending on the type of surgery recommended, as well as the health and age of the patient, families should question whether there are other options. You also can refuse surgery.

This can be a difficult conversation with medical staff. Because the business of surgeons is to perform surgery, many are reluctant to discuss nonsurgical options. A family physician can be of help in exploring alternatives. You may also want to get a second opinion from another surgeon.

If possible, don't schedule surgery right before a weekend, near major holidays, or in the afternoon. Like the rest of us, surgeons enjoy leisure time over weekends and take vacations during holiday seasons. These are times when your family won't be able to discuss complications or aftercare with the physician who performed the surgery. Although other doctors may be assigned to your patient's follow-up (in the hospital or on-call colleagues in the surgery practice), these physicians have no personal knowledge of the patient and need to rely on computer entries.

In our experience, not only are many doctors on vacation during the holidays, but office hours are reduced, on-call physicians are difficult to reach (in our case, several never returned phone calls), and hospital staff are busy and overworked.

A recent study[*] found patients whose surgery began between 3:00 p.m. and 4:00 p.m. had a higher rate of nausea, vomiting, and postoperative pain. One possible cause was a dip in circadian rhythms between 3:00 p.m. and 5:00 p.m. each day, causing sleepiness in medical staff. Another factor cited was the 3:00 p.m. shift change in surgical assistants (nurses, surgery techs, and anesthesiologists). During shift changes, key patient details may not be transmitted, or there can be delays in lab results, operating room readiness, or in-hospital transport to those rooms.

Bring the patient's insurance card(s) and medical information. The hospital or clinic will need the name, address, and phone number of the patient's primary physician, your preferred pharmacy and its address and phone number, and a list of all medications (strength and dosage). Sometimes it's easier to bring the patient's bottles of medicine, which include some of the above information, but the hospital can't dispense from your bottles. Instead, it will use its own pharmacy.

---

[*] Dr. Anthony Youn, CNN Special, citing a 2017 Duke University study.

Advice for the Waiting Room

Depending on the length of surgery, bring enough food and bottled water for yourself or money to buy those at the hospital's cafeteria or vending machines. You will also need money for parking. Think of what you will need while you wait: cell phones and chargers (although coverage is spotty in many hospital locations), crossword puzzles, knitting, iPads with video games, laptops, magazines or books, and your own medications. Most waiting rooms have comfortable furniture, but temperatures can vary, so a sweater or jacket may be needed.

After Surgery

Our family has experienced many surgeries, ranging from minor to major, and from outpatient to those requiring weeks of recuperation in a hospital. It was only recently that we learned a critical piece of information from a sympathetic nurse: every hour of surgical anesthesia takes about a month to be eliminated from the body. That is, anesthesia from a one-hour surgical procedure will take one month to clear; anesthesia from a two-hour surgery will take two months, and so on.

It would have been helpful to know this information from the start. It explains why our loved ones continued to feel dizzy, nauseated, and exhausted even weeks after surgery. The anesthesia after-effects also explained why we weren't quite tuned in after returning to work, experiencing lapses in memory and trouble with thinking and communicating. Be aware of these, and be patient with your patient.

When the surgery is completed, the patient usually goes to a recovery room for monitoring or until the anesthesia wears off. Depending on the type of surgery, the next step may be discharge from the hospital to go home;* being moved to a room in another part of the hospital for an overnight or longer stay; or referral to a rehabilitation facility for more care, either as an inpatient or outpatient.

Making the decision on where the patient goes after hospitalization is a time when the family may need to take a stronger role than it has in the past.

Patients, families, and medical staff may disagree on where to go for follow-up care.

Patients are usually eager to get back to a familiar home environment, but this may not be a realistic option (see next section, AFTERCARE). Family and friends may not be able to provide around-the-clock help or have the medical skills a patient requires after surgery (e.g., changing catheters, caring for wounds and preventing infections, or physical therapy). We found that patients were much more likely to accept a <u>doctor's</u> referral to a rehabilitation

---

* Surgery, anesthesia, and pain medications can cause patients to be weak, groggy, or nauseated. Keep plastic bags, paper towels, and wet wipes in your car so you'll be prepared for the car trip.

or step-down facility rather than taking that suggestion from family members.

Important decisions regarding a loved one can bring a family together in a crisis or can lead to arguments, guilt and blame. The ideal decision-making process is one where family members can reach consensus and inform the patient of their decision as a united front.

Each family has its own history and long-standing dynamics. Some relatives have more power or are the patient's favorites. Don't let the historically bossy aunt who lives out of town take over the discussion on aftercare. Don't let the patient's spouse, who may be overtired and overwhelmed, agree out of guilt to take the patient home directly after surgery without significant support from other family members and friends. Finances are always a consideration, but writing a check is not equal to being responsible for 24-7 care. I know of some families who have called in an objective third party, such as an attorney, to help moderate this discussion.

The following section, AFTERCARE, lists options and some things to consider when making this decision.

AFTERCARE

AFTER THE HOSPITAL stay, your medical team will recommend follow-up care for the patient. These choices, and the pros and cons of each, are discussed below.

Home Care

Be very cautious before choosing the home-care option. Most family members are exhausted by the back-and-forth trips to the hospital, the tedium of sitting in patient rooms, and the general upheaval in normal activities caused by a hospital stay. Most patients want desperately to come home after a hospital stay or surgery, rather than go to yet another medical facility.

The biggest consideration before bringing the patient home from the hospital is:

Can your family members provide the required medical care in a home setting? Is a family member or friend with medical training available to help? Many patients leave the hospital with surgical dressings (bandages), catheters or drainage tubes, monitoring equipment, new orthopedic equipment (walkers, canes, or wheelchairs), or additional medications with unknown side effects for your patient.

Is the family comfortable and competent to change surgical dressings, flush out drainage tubes, change the patient's underwear (if needed), bathe the patient, monitor blood pressure or glucose levels, and keep up with daily medications and side effects? If your family is fortunate to have someone with medical training, will this person be available 24-7 to assist?

Many patients are weak and woozy after surgery, or at least have some physical after-effects of the hospital stay. Is the caregiver able to lift and move the patient or assist with trips to the bathroom, if needed? Are there enough family members or neighbors to help with preparing meals, filling prescriptions, staying overnight with the patient, or transporting to follow-up appointments?

If the answer to any of the above questions is no, relatives alone cannot safely care for the patient at home.

I know of many instances where well-meaning family members caved in to the patient's wish to come home but soon found themselves overwhelmed and exhausted with all that was required of them. Home care can cause family tension: some family members are more willing and available than others to help out with day-to-day patient care, to take a shift, to run errands, etc.

This is a time to be compassionate but firm with a loved one who begs to come home directly from the hospital: "We want you to be safe and to heal, but we can't care for you at home until you're healthier." A united front from family members is essential in making this work.

Home-Based Nursing or Therapeutic Services

As an alternative to a rehabilitation or assisted-living center, health professionals may recommend home care supplemented by medical specialists. Some care may be covered by Medicare plans or private insurance, but families should check coverage before agreeing to home-health services.

Frequency of Home Visits by the Healthcare Professional

Depending on the type of care required, three times a week may not be enough for the skilled care the patient requires. In our family's experience, one visiting nurse failed to clean the postsurgical drainage tubes adequately, and the patient wound up getting an infection and returning to the hospital.

On the other hand, three visits per week may be just right for visits from a physical therapist.

Families should contact the referring doctor or the providing agency to request changes in a schedule if it doesn't seem to be working for the patient.

Closely observe all healthcare providers when they are in your home. Watching the patient receive care can teach family members the appropriate medical techniques, and monitoring what's happening can lead to a greater understanding of the patient's condition and treatment. In cases of speech, occupational or physical rehabilitation, therapists may recommend that the patient continue to practice certain activities or exercises several times a day, which will require encouragement and help from family members.

One of our caregivers was supposedly certified in helping patients bathe, but when we watched her, she had no idea how to lift the patient into the shower, creating a dangerous situation for the patient and herself. We immediately called the agency, who assigned someone else.

In addition, it's just good sense to keep an eye on any professional entering your home to keep the patient safe and your belongings secure.

Keep a notebook of the dates and times of service as well as the contact information for all home providers. This information may be important if there is a dispute on the bill, or if you need to get in touch with the home healthcare professional.

Nonmedical Home-Based Care

With input from the patient's physician, families should have a serious discussion about whether the patient is safe living alone. If not, the options may be hiring a home-care professional or moving to an assisted-living facility. We learned patients are more likely to accept advice from their doctor than from relatives, and our family often asked doctors for help in having this discussion with the patient.

Many patients don't require skilled nursing care in their homes, but may need companionship and daily help with household chores and errands, getting in and out of bed, using the bathroom, administering medication, monitoring blood pressure, or preparing meals.

The industry of home-care workers has grown dramatically over the past decade. Many family members live too far away from patients to visit regularly. Even family members who live with the patient may not be able to manage the double jobs of caring for the patient and keeping the household running smoothly.

A major barrier to successful home-based care may be the patient you're trying to help. Older people often are reluctant to have a stranger present in their home, especially a stranger who's unfamiliar with the routine, or doesn't do something "the way we do." In our family's experience, elderly family members have driven off many perfectly adequate home-care providers because they resented the intrusion. My mother would lock the front door and sneak out the back when she saw the care provider's car pull in the driveway.

Consider hiring a relative or friend as the home-care provider. Hiring someone you know, a person who is able to do the tasks required for the patient and the household, is ideal. The patient will feel more comfortable with a friend, neighbor, or loved one, and this may eliminate the dangers of theft and patient abuse or neglect. One group of siblings actually paid a sister to care for their mother. The sister was more than willing to provide the care, she needed the money, and everyone trusted her to look after Mom. By contributing to her salary, other family members felt less guilty about their inability or unwillingness to help.

If this option isn't available, work with an established agency to find a home-care professional.

Look for an agency with lots of home-care professionals and a history of providing this care. These agencies will have letters of recommendation from other families and may give you a list of families they have served whom you can contact. Good agencies will be licensed and bonded. Their staff will have training and certificates in health, safety, and providing home care.

Our family worked with more than twenty providers from one agency for more than a year. After talking with others and doing our research, we decided this was the best agency in our region, and we continue to recommend them to others. Their pay scale for their providers was considerably higher than other that of other agencies—a good sign, since it reduces staff turnover.

Nevertheless, here are some things we learned:

Observe the caregivers. If possible, have a relative or friend present for the first few days of care. This will tell you a lot: Do the caregivers interact in a friendly way with the patient? Do they frequently wash their hands? Can the caregivers understand instructions to perform the required tasks (e.g., operate the washing machine or vacuum, take blood pressure readings, feed the pets)? Do they take initiative or need constant reminders on what to do?

"Chemistry" is important. We found that caregivers' rapport with our patients was the deciding factor in success.

We had several caregivers who may have been perfectly competent, but their personalities just didn't work for our patient. We needed someone to engage him in conversation, someone with a sense of humor, and someone willing to cajole him into doing his physical therapy or eating healthy food. At our request, the agency removed these caregivers and reassigned to us people who had these qualities.

We had one caregiver who was cheerful and friendly and introduced new activities and games each day for our patient. In chatting with her, we discovered that her supposed training in home health care was limited to her history of caring for her sick father. She had no additional training or certification. When we reported this to the agency, they admitted that she didn't yet have a certificate but was working toward one. Because of her personality and extra efforts for our patient, however, we decided not to request reassignment.

Move your valuables off site. Unfortunately, we had caregivers who stole jewelry and medications. These were substitute staff for our regular caregivers, and the thefts occurred long before we noticed them, so we were unable to identify with certainty who took what. In retrospect, we should have moved all valuables, including unused checks and financial statements, somewhere else or kept them in a locked safe.

Accept that things will break. Even though this happens in most households on a regular basis, somehow it feels more annoying when a nonrelative breaks something. Warning: There will be knives dropped down the garbage disposal, someone will put your Teflon pans in the dishwasher, and Aunt Minnie's teacup will fall and smash. If those things are important to you, put them away.

Rehabilitation Facilities

The hospital may recommend that the patient enter a rehabilitation facility for a certain amount of time rather than go directly home.

These places are usually set up for short-term care, rather than extended stays.

Hospitals usually give families a list of rehab centers to which they refer patients. Be wary of brochures on these centers, which will contain cheerful photos, smiling staff and patients, and well-tended lawns and gardens. Your state or county may have a rating system for rehab centers, but in our experience, the worst imaginable facility we used was rated the highest: five stars.

What matters most for your patient is the quality of care in a rehabilitation facility. Ask friends about their experiences (both good and bad) and check your state Health Department's website for complaints and incident reports.

Don't sign a long-term agreement until your patient has resided there for a few months. Unfortunately, families may not be able to determine whether the facility is a good one until after the patient is admitted. If the match is not a good one, you can leave if you've signed a contract that allows that flexibility.

Here are some things to do and watch for when selecting a rehab center:

If possible, visit the rehabilitation center before moving the patient there.

Where are the patients? What are they doing? If the answers are "in their rooms" and "watching TV or sleeping," it may indicate more of a warehouse than a therapeutic facility. In one rehab center, patients in wheelchairs were lined up in the halls for hours, ignored by staff and staring at walls, until their daily hour of therapy.

It's a good sign if patients are out and about: walking the halls, in therapy rooms, socializing in a commons area, or playing cards or board games. Interacting, not just passively watching TV.

You should ask to see a sample therapy schedule and discuss with the referring hospital staff or your doctor whether it's enough to justify a stay in a center as opposed to having a physical therapist come to your home.

Ask about family participation in the therapy. We were surprised to learn that one rehab facility requested that a family member be present at all therapy sessions two or three times a day each weekday. We didn't anticipate this major commitment of time. Depending on the location of the facility, it may not be possible for families to participate at this level.

Pay attention to support staff. Keep in mind that housekeepers and techs are among the lowest-paid professionals. They perform tasks that most of us are unwilling to do. They may come from other countries and speak with heavy accents. With that said, their work will make your patient's stay either clean and comfortable, or miserable.

Is the support staff friendly to visitors and patients? When a patient's call button lights up, do they respond quickly? Are they visible in the halls or patient rooms? On the other hand, if the staff is surly, congregating in groups with each other, and not interacting with patients, this is a red flag that your loved one's care could suffer.

Is the facility clean? Look at the floors, hallways, wastebaskets, bathrooms, and day rooms to see if they meet your standards for a safe and sanitary environment.

Once again, families should be clear about goals for the patient, how progress will be measured, and what will be required before getting released. The same questions recommended for hospital stays also apply to rehab centers:

Which physician is primarily responsible for the patient's care? You should add this information to your notebook with the names and contact information of all healthcare personnel working with your patient.

What is required for the patient to leave?

Assisted Living

Moving to an assisted-living facility is a significant upheaval for both the patient and family. It is a major life event, which signifies the patient is no longer able to care for himself or herself and that the family does not have the ability to provide that care. Patients have lost control of their lives. The family dynamic has changed forever, and things will never again return to what they were in the past.

A move to assisted living can trigger grief, sadness, and anger among all parties involved. Patients may react in different but understandable ways: lashing out at relatives and caregivers, refusing to participate in social activities, insisting that their stay will be brief, or even walking away from the facility without authorization or supervision. Families may be guilt-ridden over their decision or angry with their loved one's stubborn behavior.

There are no easy answers to these dilemmas except to say that, in time, things usually calm down, and everyone settles in, however reluctantly, to this new life.

Sometime in the last decade or so, the term *assisted-living facility* has replaced the dreaded term *nursing home*. These centers often have a sister building nearby that provides inpatient residential care, now called *memory care*, for people with dementia or Alzheimer's disease.

We are fortunate that the days of housing our elderly or economically disadvantaged folks in dark unsanitary warehouses are disappearing. At the same time, however, these newer more humane facilities are not without some problems of their own.

Below are some considerations when selecting an assisted-living facility for your loved one.

Cost of Care

Your patient may have purchased long-term care insurance, but most families do not have this coverage. Union members and veterans should explore benefits through their organizations. The assisted-living facility has staff to discuss payment options, which range from a monthly fee to a contract that guarantees lifelong care (including memory care and hospice) if the patient pays up front, or surrenders some or all financial assets to the facility at death.

Medicaid, Medicare, or private insurance may cover some or all the costs of prescriptions or special nursing care associated with a patient's stay in assisted living. Policies and eligibility are different for each patient, so families should understand what is available to supplement your patient's cost of care.

There is some relationship between the cost of care and the quality of care, although it's not necessarily true that the more-expensive assisted-living facilities are the best for your patient.

You should base that decision on your visits to and observation of the facility as you did with rehabilitation facilities.

Where are the residents? What are they doing? We visited one highly regarded assisted-living facility, which appeared to have all the bells and whistles we were seeking:

a swimming pool for residents, a well-stocked library, lovely grounds with flowers and bird feeders, a gift shop, and a beautiful reception area for its five-hundred-plus residents.

Both times we toured the facility, however, we saw almost no residents in the library or commons area. No one was sitting outside or using the pool. The halls were empty, and without exception, patient doors were closed. To us, this signaled isolation of residents, a lack of activities to encourage socialization, and a facility designed to <u>look</u> good without the programming to <u>be</u> good.

We wanted to see patients out of their rooms, walking the halls, talking to each other in small informal groups, or participating in group activities like crafts, Trivial Pursuit, or listening to a guest speaker.

When we entered the lobby of another highly touted assisted-living facility, it was filled with people waiting to take a bus to a museum. Good sign. At the same time, there was an overwhelming smell of feces, indicating that the staff hadn't adequately prepared at least one resident for the trip.

Our family has had loved ones in four assisted-living facilities. We began with some research on the internet (often misleading), visited each facility several times, talked with others who had relatives living there, and finally made a decision based more on the feel of the place than on any of the publicized ratings. When possible, we included the patient as much as we could in the decision.

Develop a friendship with the staff who are assigned to your patient. While this may seem unnecessary, remember that these are the people who can make your loved one's stay cheerful and comfortable. Families cannot be there to monitor care around the clock, and patients may not be able to advocate for themselves. A good relationship with staff is particularly important if your loved one is depressed, withdrawn, angry, or even verbally abusive to others.

As explained in a previous section, these support staff are among the lowest-paid workers in the healthcare system. They perform jobs many of us are unwilling to do. They may come from other countries. English may be their second language. Every day, they have to accommodate surly, argumentative, and even combative patients while providing the most intimate of bodily care.

Learn their names. Ask for information on your loved one's progress and any difficulties they're having with the required care. Bring them small gifts (homemade baked goods, a box of doughnuts, a bag of snacks, a gift card, or an occasional cash tip, even though the facility may have rules against that)—anything to let them know that you appreciate their work. This will help set you apart from other families and could mean the difference between minimal care and special attention for your loved one.

One friend hung a large photograph of her father in his room at the assisted-living facility. It showed him as an active middle-aged man, engaged in one of his favorite activities: fly-fishing. She did this to remind caregivers and visitors that while he was now sick and elderly, he was once as vital and active as they are.

On several occasions, it became clear that the match between our family member and his caregiver was not working. Often, it was our relative who complained, but just watching the daily interaction gave us enough information to request a change in staffing from the facility manager, who was more than willing to comply with our wishes.

Visit often and at different times of the day. Our family was fortunate to have someone visit our loved ones nearly every day. We were able to talk regularly with the direct-care staff and the nurses and receptionist and to observe the meals, activities, and comings and goings of the place.

We discussed all concerns with the manager. These included changes in how medication was dispensed; vacancies in the nursing staff, which required a lot of overtime and resulted in overtired nurses; and changes to the daily menu, which upset some of the residents. Each of these concerns was successfully addressed.

Neglect and Abuse

Recent studies indicate that neglect and abuse of residents in nursing homes and assisted-care facilities are more common than previously known. Despite state laws, abuse and neglect often are not reported, or are underreported by staff.

Some instances of neglect and abuse are obvious: bed sores, visible bruises, untreated skin wounds or rashes, dirty bed linens, or signs the resident has not been bathed or cleaned in days. These should be reported immediately to the facility manager, nursing staff, and the state Health Department.

Because of close living quarters and shared commons areas, occasional outbreaks of urinary tract infections (UTIs), flu or pneumonia, and even staph infections do happen. Good facilities will inform patients and families of these conditions and take aggressive measures to isolate residents or bring in nursing and infectious-disease specialists to provide care.

Families and visitors should pay attention to the resident's physical and mental well-being during visits. If the resident feels hot to the touch, has a stomach ache, or reports any pain, you should contact the assigned staff member and nurse, who will monitor the resident for infections, bowel blockages, dehydration. Follow up to ensure the patient is better.

Residents in assisted care can become noncommunicative. Causes of this can be physical or psychological. Patients may feel abandoned, isolated, or angry at being there. Discuss your concerns with the nursing and care staff. The explanation could be as simple as a UTI, in which case an antibiotic will quickly solve the problem. If the cause is depression, fairly common in long-term care facilities, the physician may prescribe an antidepressant or activities to boost the patient's mood.

FAMILY MEMBERS, FRIENDS, AND NEIGHBORS

MEDICAL EMERGENCIES CAN create chaos for families. Most of us have limited experience with emergency rooms, hospitals, rehab or assisted-living facilities, dealing with healthcare staff, or understanding medical terminology. Even though they're under stress, families must make multiple decisions on short notice, from visiting schedules to financial and legal concerns to aftercare.

Healthcare has made almost unbelievable strides in the past century. At the same time, it may actually have been easier back then to care for sick family members. Families were larger and often lived close to each other. Patients were kept at home with multiple caregivers available to help with various tasks. Everyone had individual skills and strengths to help with patient care, and it was likely each family had members with experience in those roles. Life expectancy was what it was, with fewer pharmaceutical interventions and heroic measures available to prolong it.

These days, family members are more likely to live far away, or at least in different cities, and there are fewer of them to help in an emergency or stay on through aftercare.

Existing family dynamics can compound this emotionally charged environment. The bossy aunt, the overwhelmed spouse, the cousin who is a licensed nurse, the son who lives far away—every family has its unique history of making decisions and who's in charge.

But on short notice, families will need to answer the following: Who is ultimately responsible for managing the patient's care? Will the patient stay at home or with a relative after the hospital stay? Who will keep track of medications, medical appointments, bills, feeding pets, and the home's upkeep when the patient can't?

Based on our family's experience, below are some suggestions on navigating these decisions.

Decide which family member has the ultimate authority for the patient's care. This decision is easier if the patient has designated someone as Medical or Healthcare Power of Attorney and Financial Power of Attorney. (See next section, LEGAL AND FINANCIAL CONCERNS.) In the absence of these legal documents, however, this question should be answered in a family discussion.

The ideal is that families reach an agreement or consensus on who's responsible. Having a united front to advocate for the patient avoids family arguments, stress, and upsetting the patient. Even though there may be disagreement at first, there should be no doubt about who has the authority to make decisions on patient care (spouse, eldest child, relative living the closest). An ideal Healthcare Power of Attorney document should list these authorized persons in priority order or grant decision-making powers to any one of several people.

You can change this decision as time progresses or circumstances change, but there should always be someone who's accepted as the one in charge.

The immediate family should add friends and neighbors to its list of caregivers. Unless there are numerous relatives available to help, you may have to find friends or neighbors to supplement care. Consider the following assignments.

Beyond the Casserole

In many cultures, bringing food to the home of a sick person is probably the first response by friends and neighbors. How many of us have seen (and added to) refrigerators already filled with ready-to-heat homemade casseroles? These gifts are appreciated and needed.

But friends and neighbors should also think about food and household supplies for the long(er) term. Soups that can be frozen, items to stock the pantry, pet food, and household goods such as paper towels and soap can save the caregiver trips to the grocery store once the patient is home.

While tangible gifts of food and supplies are welcome and useful, also consider asking friends and neighbors to volunteer for other duties.

Helping with Medications

Multiple medications can be confusing to patients and caregivers.

A medication organizer, available at most pharmacies and online, helps sort medications into days of the week and times of the day when they should be given.

If possible, you should designate <u>one person</u> to be responsible for medications: discussions with the pharmacist, picking up refills, loading pills into the medication organizer each week. It goes without saying that this person should have good eyesight, hand-eye coordination, and be organized. Pills can be small, may look alike, and are clumsy to handle. Aunt Millie with liver spots on her shaky hands isn't the person for the job.

Mail, Pets, and Housekeeping

In a medical crisis, daily household routines get neglected. Mail will be piled up in different places. Pets, already aware that something is wrong, may be even more upset with the changes in their daily schedules of walking and feeding.

I suggest choosing one family member, friend or neighbor to sort the mail into bills and important letters (e.g., from the insurance company or Medicare); if possible, assign one person to pay bills and write checks.

Someone or a group of people should be solely responsible for feeding and walking pets on a schedule that's as close to their usual routine as possible.

Obviously, you'll want to ask someone who is reliable and trustworthy since you'll be giving them access to your home and valuables.

Dirty dishes, unwashed laundry, and overgrown lawns can be upsetting for the patient or caregiver. While these household chores may not directly affect good patient care, they do affect the healing environment and caregiver stress. If friends, family members, or neighbors aren't available to help, consider hiring an agency for home and lawn care. Stay home to supervise the work of these outsiders.

Give Caregivers a Break

Speaking from personal experience, caregivers may be unwilling to accept help. To stay physically and emotionally healthy, caregivers need an occasional change in their routine. A meal out, a weekend vacation, or even a few free hours in the day while someone else monitors patient care offer caregivers the short breaks they need.

LEGAL AND FINANCIAL CONCERNS

SICKNESS AND DEATH are difficult topics for family discussions. We avoid making plans until medical emergencies happen. By then, it's often too late to find out the patient's wishes regarding care and end-of-life choices.

Fortunately, there are legal documents to help families make financial and healthcare decisions before a crisis. Outlines or templates of these documents are available online, so you can complete them by yourself without involving an attorney or outside professional.

In our experience, however, it's always better to meet with an attorney to formalize these documents. Lawyers have the skills to guide these family discussions, playing the role of objective third-party adviser on what can be emotional decisions, and asking questions you hadn't considered. There might be state laws and requirements that the template documents available on the internet don't cover. You can also use the appointment with an attorney to update wills and other financial documents.

Give copies of all legal and financial documents to all named or involved people. In an emergency, you want to have the paperwork needed to make decisions. Plan ahead and keep these documents in a safe place you'll remember when you're under duress. You don't want to be calling your attorney, or an out-of-state brother in the middle of the night to send you a copy of the patient's Medical Power of Attorney.

The following pages describe some of the legal and financial documents to discuss with your attorney.

<u>Medical Power of Attorney (Also Called Power of Attorney for Healthcare or Durable Power of Attorney for Healthcare)</u>

This document is used when the patient (family member) is too ill or incapacitated to make those decisions.

The Medical POA can be one person or several people. For example, my mother designated all four of her children to have Medical POA, but only one of their signatures was required to authorize her health care at all stages of her illness. We all lived in different cities, so this prevented having to get all four of our signatures before a decision could be made.

Other families put the Medical POA names in priority order. For instance, the wife is named as the primary decision-maker, but if she is unavailable or incapacitated, the POA might list the child who lives closest, then the eldest child, then a sister—in that order. To repeat: Get these documents done and distributed to all parties before you need them.

<u>Living Will (Also Known as Advanced Healthcare Directive)</u>

This document is a person's end-of-life instructions to healthcare providers. It directs physicians not to use artificial means or heroic measures to keep the patient alive if there is no chance of recovery and death is likely to occur within a relatively short time. It defines "terminal condition" in accordance with your state's laws. The Living Will also authorizes the physician to issue Do Not Resuscitate (DNR) orders if certain conditions are met.

Hospitals and doctors' offices will ask if the patient has a living will. Having one will make it easier for them and the family to make informed clinical decisions that take into account the patient's wishes.

Financial Power of Attorney

This is similar to the Medical Power of Attorney, but it names the person or people empowered to make financial and other legal decisions on the patient's behalf. This POA requires a different skill set from making healthcare decisions. Your family may be fortunate enough to have a banker, accountant, or economist, or to know someone who would be willing to take on this responsibility. If not, your lawyer may have a recommendation.

Guardianship

Guardianship allows another person to make financial and legal decisions when someone is incapacitated and unable to handle those matters autonomously. Guardians are appointed and supervised by a court judge.

While this may seem like a good option, families should be wary. First, judges must approve every expenditure for or on behalf of the patient, even the smallest of financial transactions. Does your family want to go through this bureaucratic process whenever a bill needs to be paid?

Recent news stories have revealed that some third-party court-appointed guardians can and do take advantage of their clients. These unscrupulous professionals can pay themselves huge fees with little or no oversight. Some have hundreds of clients, who may wind up in long-term care facilities, neglected with no monitoring or advocacy on their behalf.

If the patient should recover, it may be very difficult to reverse the court's guardianship appointment.

Will

It is never too early to hire an attorney to draft your will. This legal document spells out how you want your assets to be distributed after your death. Wills can always be written or rewritten to accommodate changes: new family members (for example, grandchildren), or new charitable interests (through a gift to a not-for-profit organization).

A good attorney can draft a will to include these future possibilities without having to return for frequent rewrites.

Medical Bills

Your health insurance and participation in Medicare or Medicaid are the first sources used for medical bills. For many patients, however, the cost of care may be greater than what's covered.

Do not ignore medical bills. We do not live in nineteenth-century Europe. You cannot be jailed if you can't pay your medical bills. Children are not responsible for their parents' medical bills.

Medical providers (physicians, hospitals, clinics, therapists) will work with patients and families to set up realistic payment schedules. I have a friend whose medical bills over the past decade added up to hundreds of thousands of dollars. She is unable to work and lives on a small fixed income below the state-poverty level for single people. She discussed her financial situation with the accounts receivable departments of her healthcare teams and was able to get approval for a relatively small monthly payment she can afford.

There is no way my friend will live long enough to cover the total costs of her treatment. The hospitals and clinics will eventually write off her debts. But her good faith efforts to contact billing offices and to keep up with regular payments have saved her from having to worry about the costs of her care.

Healthcare providers will negotiate a fair payment plan **if you contact them**. No response from you will put your outstanding medical bills in the hands of a for-profit credit company. These companies can be ruthless in pursuing payment, threatening prosecution and garnishment of wages, adding undue stress to an already-difficult situation.

SUMMARY

An unexpected medical crisis can bring out the best and the worst in family dynamics. Important decisions must be made quickly and under stressful conditions. Families may not have a clear understanding of the patient's wishes—either because those conversations were never held during healthy times, or the legal documents that could clarify those wishes may not exist.

I want to assure you that you ARE in control. However inexperienced families may be with healthcare settings and providers, you can and should play a major role in determining the best course of care for your loved one.

Here are some things to remember:

Find the Best Environment for Your Patient to Heal. Remember that hospitals and aftercare facilities are businesses. Whether they are for-profit or not-for-profit organizations, hospitals must make good financial decisions if they are to keep their doors open. They must work closely with public and private insurance companies to assure expenses will be covered. They must avoid expensive medical liability lawsuits to remain solvent. When we understand those constraints, it's clear that the physical well-being of our patient may not be their top priority.

Families have more leverage than they may realize to find the best medical setting for the patient. Get a clear understanding of the objectives of the hospital stay: what needs to be accomplished, and how it will be measured so that the patient can be discharged or transferred. If aftercare is warranted, make sure your decision is as well-informed as it can be. Beware of bringing patients home prematurely if the family isn't prepared to provide medical assistance. Stay involved and informed in every medical environment.

Develop Partnerships and Friendships with Healthcare Staff. Families are understandably reluctant to ask questions of healthcare staff. It's hard to admit they don't understand the diagnosis, medications, or course of treatment. Busy medical settings and overworked staff are not conducive to long, leisurely conversations.

That said, healthcare staff chose their profession because of a desire to help people. If treated as the professionals they are, they will welcome informed and engaged families. Most are willing to provide assistance and explanations if they are treated with respect and courtesy.

If you are not getting the quality of health care your patient needs, you should request a change in the assigned staff.

Maintain Presence and Control. The welfare of critically ill patients cannot be handed off to insurance companies or healthcare providers. The patient's family and friends must stay involved at every step of the patient's hospitalization and aftercare. If family and friends are unavailable, consider hiring a private patient advocate to fulfill these duties.

This means frequent visits to get updates on the course of treatment and to observe how the patient is progressing, staying on top of medications and potential medication drift, ensuring that accurate records follow the patient if transferring to another facility, keeping good records of meetings with healthcare staff, and making sure everyone has copies of the patient's legal documents.

Reach Out to Others for Help. Don't wait until the patient's primary caregiver is overwhelmed and exhausted before asking extended family members and neighbors for their help. Most people are more than willing, but they need specific assignments. These can be patient-centered (hospital visits, transportation to medical appointments) or jobs that keep things running smoothly at home (collecting mail, paying bills, feeding pets).

My Thanks

This book reflects twenty years of our family's and friends' experiences with navigating and working in the healthcare system. I'm grateful to the many generous relatives and friends who allowed me to include their personal histories and suggestions in this book.

ABOUT THE AUTHOR

PEGGY CALESTRO WROTE this handbook to provide advice to families and friends of hospitalized patients. The book is a compilation of her friends' and family's experiences, both as patients and practitioners in the healthcare system.

Peggy's professional career was in education and philanthropy, where she developed and administered a variety of programs to improve lives. She and her daughter coauthored *Lost and Found in Appalachia*. She lives in Columbus, Ohio.

CPSIA information can be obtained
at www.ICGtesting.com
Printed in the USA
LVHW110153291220
675313LV00008B/110